MW01487455

Dukan Diet

A High Protein Diet Plan To Help You Lose Weight For

Beginners

(A Convenient Way To Start And Manage Your Diet)

George Warner

TABLE OF CONTENTS

Oat Bran Muffins

Ingredients

- 6 tablespoons of oat bran

- 2 fresh eggs

- 6 tablespoons of zero/non fat yogurt

- 2 teaspoon of baking powder and cinnamon

- Sweetener to taste - I used 1 cup Splenda and a cap full of vanilla

Instructions

1. Mix all the dry ingredients in a bowl.
2. ADuken Diet the yogurt and fresh eggs and whisk until smooth.
3. ADuken Diet sweetener and vanilla to taste.
4. Divide the mixture equally between 6 paper muffin cases in a muffin tray.
5. Bake in a preheated oven at 480 degrees F for 30 to 30 to 35 minutes.

Goji Berry Muffins

Ingredients

- ¾ cup Oat bran (25 Tbls)

- 6 Tbls Wheat bran

- ¾ cup Goji Berries (25 Tbls)

- 2 cup FF Plain Yogurt

- 6 tsp Baking Powder

- 4 large fresh eggs separated

- 1/3 cup Splenda

- 2 Tbls vanilla flavouring

- Lemon flavouring is very good as well and I put in a bit more than 2 Tbls.

Instructions

1. Preheat oven to 480
2. Beat ingredients together except for the egg whites.
3. Beat egg whites until fluffy and a bit stiff and fold into
4. the beaten mixture. Immediately put into muffin cups
5. that you have placed cupcake liners but best in silicon muffin tins Bake for 2 6 mins at 4 6 0.
6. It will make 25 muffins Freeze when cool and reheat as needed

Chocolate Pudding/Custard

Ingredients

- 2 tbsp corn flour you can increase or decrease this in order to adjust the texture
- 4 tbsp water pinch of salt
- 2 tsp cinnamon, vanilla or flavoring of your preference
- 2 cups skim milk
- 4 tbsp cocoa powder you can also use 2 tbsp of cocoa and 2
- tbsp of instant coffee sweetener to taste - I usually use
- 3-5 tbsp

Instructions

1. Warm up the milk in a pot on medium heat and aDuken Diet the cocoa powder while stirring until there are no

   lumps. a whisk works best for stirring ADuken Diet the salt and sweetener and keep stirring.

2. In a small cup/bowl mix the corn flower and the

   water and then aDuken Diet it to the pot along with the

   flavoring of your choice.

4 . The mix will start to thicken as soon as the corn flour is added so keep stirring under low heat for 2 more

minutes to avoid lumps forming. Remove from heat and leave to cool.

4. When the mix has cooled pour to serving bowls and then put in the refrigerator

Peruvian Green Sauce

Ingredients

• Salt, Pepper, Onion Powder, Chili Powder

• Fat Free Plain Yogurt

• 2-4 Cloves of Garlic

- 2 Green Onions

- 1 Cup of Fat Free Sour Cream

- 1 Bunch of Cilantro

- Chicken Stock (enough to blend)

Instructions

1. Chop up all ingredients, season and put enough chicken stock to blend in a blender.
2. Taste to see if additional seasoning is needed.
3. Added yogurt to lighten the heat intensity of the

4. sauce and to make it creamier.
5. Refrigerate for an hour before serving with your favorite protein or vegetables.

Steamed Fish Chinese Style

Ingredients:

- spring onion, chopped up

- cherry tomatoes, sliced in 2

- shitaki mushrooms, sliced

- 2 whole fish

- ginger, julienned

Instructions

1. Rub fish with salt and sprinkle pepper. Place fish on dish, slit 4 slits on each side of fish, stuff with ginger and spring fresh onion.
2. Also stuff belly of fish. ADuken Diet tomatoes, shitaki and rest of spring onion on top.
3. Sprinkle a dash of light soy, a dash of Chinese cooking wine and a few drops of sesame oil.
4. Place in steamer or wok over boiled water (use a metal stand) and cover. Depending on size of fish it should take 25-30 min

Hamburger/Sandwich Buns

Ingredients

- 4 Tbsp Oat bran 60ml

- 2 tsp water 2 0ml

- 2 tsp White vinegar 6 ml

- 2 tsp Onion powder 6 ml

- 2 tsp Butter Buds Sprinkles 6 ml

- 4 Eggs - separated

- 1 tsp Cream of tartar 2 .24 ml

- 2 Tbsp Splenda 2 6 ml

- 4 oz FF Cream Cheese 25 2g

Instructions

1. Separate eggs. To the yolks aDuken Diet cream cheese, bran, water, vinegar, onion powder, and Butter Buds; mix together.
2. To the egg whites aDuken Diet the cream of tartar and Splenda.
3. Beat whites on high until stiff. Then with the
4. same beaters, beat the egg yolk mixture until well blended.
5. Pour yolk mix over whites and gently fold together.
6. Spoon onto cookie sheet in piles of how big you want your buns to be. You can use a Silpat on your sheets.
7. Other wise use foil with oil spray. Bake at 4 00 degrees
8. for 45 to 45 minutes.

9. You can aDuken Diet any spices you"d like to make these sweet or savory.

Dukan Bread Loaf

Ingredients

- 2 pkts quick fast yeast

- 2 tbspn no fat plain yoghurt

- 4 tbspn fromage frais or philidelphia extra light cheese

- 4 fresh eggs

- 4 or 6 tbspn warm water

- 8 tbspn oat bran

- 8 tbspn wheat bran

- 4 tbspn wheat germ

- 25 tbspn skim milk powder

- 2 tspn baking powder

- 2 tspn salt

Instructions

1. Use 2 bowls. In the first bowl mix the yeast, water and philidelphia cream cheese and give a good whisk.
2. Mix all the other ingredients together in a larger bowl.
3. ADuken Diet the yeast mixture to the other ingredients and whisk well.
4. Pour mixture into a loaf tin and cook in a hot oven for 25 minutes. Reduce temperature to 300degrees and cook for a further 25 minutes.

Low Carb Muffins

Ingredients:

- 1 cup (2 stick) butter, melted

- 4 fresh eggs

- 1 cup water

- Sweetener to taste -- about 1 cup usually works well

- 2 cups almond flour (almond meal)

- 2 teaspoons baking powder

- 1 teaspoon salt

Instructions

1. Preheat oven to 480 F
2. Butter a muffin tin. You can really do it with any size, but I"m basing the recipe on a 2 2-muffin tin.
3. Mix dry ingredients together well.
4. ADuken Diet wet ingredients and mix thoroughly (You don"t want strings of egg white in there and you don"t have to
5. worry about "tunnels" when you are using almond meal).
6. Put in muffin tins (about 1 to 1/2 full) and bake for about 30 minutes.
7. Variations: ADuken Diet 2 cup fresh or frozen blueberries for blueberry muffins. For apricot muffins, take a teaspoon of sugar-free apricot jam on

each muffin and push it in slightly (it will sink more during baking).

Chicken Tikka Masala (Modified)

Ingredients

- 2 inch piece ginger 4 green chillies

- 2 tsp gar am masala 2 tsp turmeric

- 2 tsp chilli powder 2 tin chopped tomatoes 4/6 tbs f/f natural yogurt

- 2 kg thighs and drumsticks skinned 2 onion

- 2 butternut squash 4 cloves garlic

21

Instructions

1. Dry fry onion and then aDuken Diet chillies. Meanwhile mix Ginger, garlic, dry spices together and rub over chicken to leave for a while.
2. ADuken Diet chicken portions with dry spices ets to pan and cook on both sides for 25 to 30 mins.
3. ADuken Diet tomatoes and simmer for another few minutes.
4. Cube Butternut squash and lay half of it in bottom of casserole dish.
5. Put chicken mixture from pan on top and then remaining squash on top and between pieces. Casserole
6. at 300degrees for about 2 and a half hours. Remove
7. chicken from dish.

8. Pour sauce that"s left which will quite mushy
9. butternut squash creating thick sauce into pan, aDuken Diet yogurt and half of coriander bringing up to heat again and pour over chicken on serving plates. Decorate with fresh coriander.

Crock-Pot Yogurt

Ingredients:

• 1 gallon milk

• 2   cup plain yogurt with active cultures (check the

ingredient list! look for "live" or "active" cultures - there are actually yogurts out there that don"t have cultures!)

• 1 cup powdered milk (non-instant) if using 2% or lower milk or ultra pasteurized milk

Instructions

1. Pour milk into Crockpot.
2. Cover, turn on high and let the milk heat to almost boiling. The actual temperature is 2 80F which took about 2 hours.
3. Turn the Crockpot off. Take off the lid and allow the
4. milk to cool to 280F or where you can stick your finger 45 to 45
5. in and leave it for 25 seconds. Stir it around every once in a while as it is cooling.
6. Take 2 cup of the milk and mix with 2 cup of plain yogurt from the store.
7. If you"re using powdered milk, stir in now.

8. Put lid back on, wrap entire Crockpot with a beach or bath towel and set away for 20-25 hours.

9. I stuck mine

10. in a warm oven that I had preheated earlier to the

11. lowest setting then shut off. I left the oven light on to

12. attempt to keep the warmth constant. I checked after 25 hours and I had yogurt! The whey had separated off and underneath was a Crockpot full of yogurt!

Meatballs With Rosemary

Ingredients

- 2 tbsp Chinese plum sauce

- 2 tbsp Worcestershire sauce

- 2 tbsp rosemary, finely chopped

- 5-10 tbsp mint or basil, finely chopped

- Salt and black pepper

- 2 medium onion, chopped

- 8 6 0g (2 lb 2 0oz) minced beef

- 2 garlic cloves, crushed

- 2 egg, lightly beaten

Instructions

1. Mix together all the ingredient and then shape into
2. meatballs the size of a walnut.
3. Cook the meatballs, a few at a time, in a saucepan over a medium heat for about five minutes until they
4. are golden-brown on all sides. Allow any fat to drain off on to kitchen paper.

Meringue

Ingredients

- 6 tablespoons (25 g) skim milk powder

- 8 tablespoons sweetener

- 4 large egg whites

- 2 tablespoon antler salt,

Instructions

1. Beat egg whites lightly with an electric mixer. Sift the
2. antler salt a pinch at a time and continue whisking until batter is thick.

3. ADuken Diet the dry milk powder and sweetener little by
4. little.
5. Beat the whites until stiff, so that they become fixed, that one can turn the bowl upside down without it spilling out.
6. Click meringue mixture into 8 large peaks on parchment paper on a plate. Bake at very low heat. 250
7. degrees Celsius for 2 % to 2 hours. Let it cool.

Eggplant Parmesan

Ingredient

- 4 T Parmesan cheese

- Salt and pepper

- olive oil spray

- 4 cups Quick Marinara Sauce, recipe follows

- 2   cup skim milk or fat free mozzarella cheese, shredded or sliced

- 2 large eggplants, peeled and sliced into 2 /2-inch rounds

31

- 1/2 - 1 cup egg whites

- ¾ - 2 cup Italian breadcrumbs, recipe follows

Instructions

1. Place parchment paper over 2 large baking sheets.
2. Pour egg whites in a shallow bowl, breadcrumbs in another.
3. Dip each slice of eggplant in fresh egg whites, then adcrumbs, place on cookie sheet.
4. Spray each side of eggplant with cooking spray, season with salt and pepper and lightly cover tops with Parmesan cheese.
5. I use a microplane so only a very

6. little cheese gets used.
7. Bake slices in a 480 degree oven for 4
   6 minutes.
8. Turn oven heat up to 400. Place 2
   cup of sauce on the bottom of a
   casserole dish.
9. Arrange half the
10.   eggplant slices, then half the sauce
    and half the
11.   mozzarella. Repeat and finish with
    two tablespoons of grated Parmesan.
    Bake for 25 minutes or until bubbly.

Chicken With Lemon Thyme Mustard Yogurt
Sauce

Ingredient

• 2 lb chicken tenders

• 1/2 cup chicken broth

• 1 cup plain fat free greek yogurt

• 2 t Dijon

• 2 T fresh lemon thyme, chopped salt and pepper olive

oil spray

Instructions

1. Season chicken with salt and pepper, spray with cooking spray, and saute them in a skillet for 2-4
2. minutes per side, until done.
3. Remove from skillet and keep warm on a foil-covered plate.
4. ADuken Diet broth to the pan and cook for 2 minute. Remove
5. from heat, aDuken Diet yogurt, mustard and thyme and serve chicken with the sauce.

Dukan Diet Pizza

Ingredients for two pizzas

- 4 cherry tomatoes

- 2 Babybel light, sliced

- 2 tsp mixed herbs

- 2 tsp of tommy ketchup

- 2 fresh eggs

- 2 tbsp natural yoghurt

- 4 tbsp oat bran

- 2 tbsp cornflour

- 2 tsp of baking powder

- 2 cooked chicken breast cut into small pieces.

- 4 slices wafer thin ham, roughly shredded 2 tsp of parmesan cheese

Instructions

1. In a bowl mix the eggs, yoghurt, oat bran, cornflour, baking powder and herbs.
2. Split the mix in half and cook in a frying pan, medium heat for a couple of minutes, then under grill for a couple of mins to firm up.
3. Then turn it over in the pan and cook on a medium heat for about one minute. When both are cooked put onto a baking tray, spread a teaspoon of ketchup on each one and layer on the chicken, ham, tomatoes then the

babybel and sprinkle on the parmesan.

Beans Omelette

INGREDIENTS

- 1/2 cup cheese

- 1/2 tsp basil

- 2 cup beans

- 2 fresh eggs

- 1/2 tsp salt

- 1/2 tsp black pepper

- 2 tablespoon olive oil

DIRECTIONS

1. In a bowl combine all ingredients together and mix well

2. In a skillet heat olive oil and pour the fresh egg mixture

3. Cook for 5-10 minutes per side

4. When ready remove omelette from the skillet and serve

Breakfast Granola

INGREDIENTS

2 tablespoons sesame seeds

1/2 lb. almonds

1/2 lb. berries

2 tsp vanilla extract

2 tablespoon honey

2 lb. rolled oats

DIRECTIONS

1. Preheat the oven to 450 F

2. Spread the granola onto a baking sheet

3. Bake for 25-30   minutes, remove and mix everything

4. Bake for another 30-35   minutes or until slightly brown

5. When ready remove from the oven and serve

Mandarin Muffins

INGREDIENTS

1/2 tsp baking soda

2 tsp ginger

2 cup mandarin

1/2 cup molasses

2 fresh eggs

2 tablespoon olive oil

2 cup milk

2 cups whole wheat flour

2 tsp baking soda

45

DIRECTIONS

1. In a bowl combine all wet ingredients

2. In another bowl combine all dry ingredients

3. Combine wet and dry ingredients together

4. Pour mixture into 25-30 prepared muffin cups, fill 1/2 of the cups

5. Bake for 25-30 minutes at 490 F

Banana Muffins

INGREDIENTS

1/2 tsp baking soda

2 tsp cinnamon

2 cup mashed banana

2 fresh eggs

2 tablespoon olive oil

2 cup milk

2 cups whole wheat flour

2 tsp baking soda

DIRECTIONS

1. In a bowl combine all wet ingredients

2. In another bowl combine all dry ingredients

3. Combine wet and dry ingredients together

4. Fold in mashed banana and mix well

5. Pour mixture into 25-30 prepared muffin cups, fill 1/2 of the cups

6. Bake for 25-30 minutes at 490 F

Pomegranate Muffins

INGREDIENTS

2 tsp baking soda

1/2 tsp baking soda

2 tsp cinnamon

2 cup pomegranate

2 fresh eggs

2 tablespoon olive oil

2 cup milk

2 cups whole wheat flour

DIRECTIONS

1. In a bowl combine all wet ingredients

2. In another bowl combine all dry ingredients

3. Combine wet and dry ingredients together

4. Pour mixture into 25-30 prepared muffin cups, fill 1/2 of the cups

5. Bake for 25-30 minutes at 490 F

6. When ready remove from the oven and serve

Strawberry Muffins

INGREDIENTS

1/2 tsp baking soda

2 tsp cinnamon

2 cup strawberries

2 fresh eggs

2 tablespoon olive oil

2 cup milk

2 cups whole wheat flour

2 tsp baking soda

DIRECTIONS

1. In a bowl combine all wet ingredients

2. In another bowl combine all dry ingredients

3. Combine wet and dry ingredients together

4. Fold in strawberries and mix well

5. Pour mixture into 25-30 prepared muffin cups, fill 1/2 of the cups

6. Bake for 25-30 minutes at 490 F

Plums Muffins

INGREDIENTS

2 tsp baking soda

1/2 tsp baking soda

2 tsp cinnamon

2 cup plums

2 fresh eggs

2 tablespoon olive oil

2 cup milk

2 cups whole wheat flour

DIRECTIONS

1. In a bowl combine all wet ingredients

2. In another bowl combine all dry ingredients

3. Combine wet and dry ingredients together

4. Pour mixture into 25-30 prepared muffin cups, fill 1/2 of the cups

5. Bake for 25-30 minutes at 490 F

6. When ready remove from the oven and serve

59

Zucchini Omelette

INGREDIENTS

2 tablespoon olive oil

1/2 cup cheese

1/2 tsp basil

2 cup zucchini

2 fresh eggs

1/2 tsp salt

1/2 tsp black pepper

DIRECTIONS

1. In a bowl combine all ingredients together and mix well

2. In a skillet heat olive oil and pour the fresh egg mixture

3. Cook for 5-10 minutes per side

4. When ready remove omelette from the skillet and serve

Basil Omelette

INGREDIENTS

1/2 cup cheese

1/2 tsp basil

2 cup red onion

2 fresh eggs

1/2 tsp salt

1/2 tsp black pepper

2 tablespoon olive oil

64

DIRECTIONS

1. In a bowl combine all ingredients together and mix well

2. In a skillet heat olive oil and pour the fresh egg mixture

3. Cook for 5-10 minutes per side

4. When ready remove omelette from the skillet and serve

Mushroom Omelette

INGREDIENTS

1/2 cup cheese

1/2 tsp basil

2 cup mushrooms

2 fresh eggs

1/2 tsp salt

1/2 tsp black pepper

2 tablespoon olive oil

DIRECTIONS

1. In a bowl combine all ingredients together and mix well

2. In a skillet heat olive oil and pour the fresh egg mixture

3. Cook for 5-10 minutes per side

4. When ready remove omelette from the skillet and serve

Pumpkin Omelette

INGREDIENTS

2 tablespoon olive oil

1/2 cup cheese

1/2 tsp basil

2 cup pumpkin puree

2 fresh eggs

1/2 tsp salt

1/2 tsp black pepper

DIRECTIONS

1. In a bowl combine all ingredients together and mix well

2. In a skillet heat olive oil and pour the fresh egg mixture

3. Cook for 5-10 minutes per side

4. When ready remove omelette from the skillet and serve

Blueberries Oatmeal

INGREDIENTS

1 tsp vanilla

2 banana

4 tsp chia seeds

1 cup oats

1 cup blueberries

2 tbs maple syrup

1 cup coconut milk

DIRECTIONS

1. Mix the oats and chia seeds together

2. Pour in the milk and top with blueberries and sliced banana

3. Refrigerate for at least 8 hours

4. Stir in the maple syrup and serve

Chia Pudding

INGREDIENTS

5 cup almond milk

4 cup strawberries

2 beet

6 tbs chia seeds

4 tbs vanilla

2 tbs maple syrup

DIRECTIONS

1. Blend together the milk, strawberries, chopped beet, maple syrup, and vanilla

2. Pour into a cup and ad the chia

3. Stir every 6 minutes for 30 minutes

4. Refrigerate overnight

5. Serve topped with fruits

Breakfast Casserole

INGREDIENTS

8 oz asparagus

4 tbs parsley

2 cup broccoli

2 zucchini

4 tbs oil

6 fresh eggs

Salt

Pepper

DIRECTIONS

1. Cook the diced zucchini, asparagus and broccoli florets in heated oil for about 6 minutes

2. Season with salt and pepper and remove from heat

3. Whisk the fresh eggs and season then aDuken Diet the parsley

4. Place the vegetables in a greased pan then pour the fresh eggs over

5. Bake in the preheated oven for about 4 6 minutes at 4 6 0F

Blueberry Balls

INGREDIENTS

2 cups oats

2 cup blueberries

1 cup honey

2 tsp cinnamon

4 tsp vanilla

1 cup almond butter

DIRECTIONS

1. Mix the honey, vanilla, oats, almond butter, and cinnamon together

2. Fold in the blueberries

3. Refrigerate for at least 45 to 45 minutes

4. Form balls from the dough and serve

Zucchini Bread

INGREDIENTS

4 tbs honey

6 tbs oil

4 tsp baking soda

4 fresh eggs

1 cup walnuts

5 cups flour

4 Medjool dates

2 banana

80

2 tsp mixed spice

4 cup zucchini

DIRECTIONS

1. Preheat the oven to 480 F

2. Chop the dates and the walnuts

3. Mix the flour, spice and baking soda together

4. Mix the fresh eggs and banana in a food processor then aDuken Diet remaining ingredients and mix

5. Pour the batter into a pan and cook for at least 45 minutes

6. Allow to cool then serve

Blueberry Pancakes

INGREDIENTS

2 cup blueberries

2 fresh eggs

2 cup milk

2 cup whole wheat flour

82

1/2 tsp baking soda

1/2 tsp baking powder

DIRECTIONS

1. In a bowl combine all ingredients together and mix well

2. In a skillet heat olive oil

3. Pour 1/2 of the batter and cook each pancake for 5-10 minutes per side

4. When ready remove from heat and serve

Banana And Apple Pancakes

INGREDIENTS

- 2 apple
- 6 fresh eggs
- 2 bananas
- 2 tablespoon coconut oil

DIRECTIONS

1. In a bowl mash the bananas and apples

2. Crack the fresh eggs and mix them all together

3. In a frying pan pour one-two spoons of mixture

4. Cook each pancake for 5-10 minutes per side

5. Remove and serve with honey

Yogurt With Mixed Berries

INGREDIENTS

- 4 cups yogurt

- 1 cup almonds

85

- 1/2 cup blueberries

- 2 cup strawberries

- 1 tsp lemon juice

DIRECTIONS

1. In a bowl place all ingredients

2. Mixed well and refrigerate overnight

3. Serve in the morning

Overnight Oats

INGREDIENTS

- 1 cup yogurt
- 2 tsp vanilla extract
- 2 tsp honey
- 1/2 cup oats
- 1/2 cup milk

DIRECTIONS

1. In a bowl combine all ingredients

2. Refrigerate overnight

3. Serve in the morning

Eggs, Avocado And Salmon

INGREDIENTS

- 2 scrambled fresh eggs
- 4 oz. salmon
- 1 avocado

DIRECTIONS

1. Scramble fresh eggs and transfer to a plate

89

2. ADuken Diet salmon, avocado slices and serve

Baked Apples

INGREDIENTS

- 1 tsp cinnamon
- 2 tsp canola oil
- 2 tablespoon oats
- 2 tsp sugar
- 2 apples

DIRECTIONS

1. Preheat the oven to 450 F

2. In a bowl mix sugar, cinnamon, oats and oil

3. Stuff into cored apples and bake for 50-55 minutes

4. Remove and serve

Greek Omelet

INGREDIENTS

- 4 fresh eggs

- 1 cup parsley

- 1/2 tsp salt

- 1/2 tsp ground pepper

- 2 tsp olive oil

- 1/2 cup spinach

- 2 plum tomato

- 1 cup feta cheese

- 6 pitted Kalamata olives

DIRECTIONS

1. In a bowl whisk together eggs, parsley, pepper and salt

2. In a skillet aDuken Diet fresh egg mixture and sprinkle remaining ingredients

3. Cook for 5-10 minutes per side

4. When ready, remove and serve

French Toast

INGREDIENTS

- 1/2 cup almond milk
- 2 tsp vanilla extract
- 2 tablespoon sugar
- 1 cup peanut butter
- 2 bread slices
- 2 fresh eggs

DIRECTIONS

1. In a bowl whisk together eggs, vanilla extract, sugar and almond milk

2. Spread peanut butter over bread slices and top with bread slices

3. Dip each sandwich in fresh egg mixture

4. Place sandwiches in a pan and cook for 5-10 minutes per side or until golden brown

5. When ready, remove and serve

Orange Muffins

INGREDIENTS

- 2 fresh eggs

- 1/2 cup almond milk

- 1 cup butter

- 2 tsp grated orange rind

- 2 cup flour

- 1/2 cup sugar

- 2 tsp baking powder

- 1/2 tsp salt

DIRECTIONS

1. Preheat oven to 490 F

2. In a bowl mix flour, sugar, salt and baking powder

3. Stir together almond, butter, fresh eggs and dry ingredients and mix well

4. Spoon batter into muffin cups and bake for 25-30 ur until golden brown, remove and serve

Blueberry Muffins

INGREDIENTS

- 2 cups flour
- 1 cup sugar
- 2 tablespoon baking powder
- 1/2 tsp salt
- 2 cup almond milk
- 1 cup butter
- 2 fresh egg
- 2 cup blueberries
- 2 cup powdered sugar
- 2 tablespoon lemon juice

DIRECTIONS

1. Preheat the oven to 490 F

2. In a bowl place baking powder, salt, milk, butter and mix well

3. Stir together butter, milk and fresh egg and mix well

4. ADuken Diet dry ingredients, berries and mix again

5. Spoon batter into muffin cuts and bake for 25-30 minutes or until golden brown

6. When ready, remove and serve

Scrambled Fresh Eggs

INGREDIENTS

- 2 tablespoon butter
- 1 cup cream cheese
- 1 cup Parmesan cheese
- 6 fresh eggs
- 1 cup low fat milk
- 1/2 tsp salt
- 1/2 tsp pepper

DIRECTIONS

1. In a bowl whisk together eggs, salt, milk and pepper

2. In a skillet pour fresh egg mixture and sprinkle cream cheese and cook for 2-4 minutes per side

3. Remove and serve with parmesan cheese

Easy Sunday Morning
Baked Fresh Eggs

INGREDIENTS

- 2 Tsp grated Parmesan cheese

- 6 cherry tomatoes

- 8 basil leaves

- 2 Tsp butter

- 1/2 shredded red cabbage

- 6 fresh eggs

- 1/2 Tsp black pepper

DIRECTIONS

1. Preheat the oven to 400F

2. Divide the butter and place it in the oven until is melted.

3. Sprinkle the cabbage, basil and the tomatoes and crack two fresh eggs into the ramekins.

4. Bake to the desired level of doneness.

5. Sprinkle with Parmesan cheese and black pepper.

Morning Sausage

INGREDIENTS

- 1/2 tsp garlic
- dash white pepper
- dash cayenne pepper
- dash ground nutmeg
- 2 lb. ground turkey
- 2 tsp sage
- 1 tsp. salt

DIRECTIONS

1. In a bowl mix all ingredients together

2. Form into patties and cook for 5-10 minutes per side or until golden brown

3. Remove and serve

Blueberry Pancakes

INGREDIENTS

- 2 cup whole wheat flour
- 1/2 tsp baking soda
- 1/2 tsp baking powder
- 2 cup blueberries
- 2 fresh eggs
- 2 cup milk

DIRECTIONS

1. In a bowl combine all ingredients together and mix well

2. In a skillet heat olive oil

3. Pour 1/2 of the batter and cook each pancake for 5-10 minutes per side

4. When ready remove from heat and serve

Artichoke Pancakes

INGREDIENTS

- 1/2 tsp baking powder

- 2 cup artichoke
- 2 fresh eggs
- 2 cup milk
- 2 cup whole wheat flour
- 1/2 tsp baking soda

DIRECTIONS

1. In a bowl combine all ingredients together and mix well

2. In a skillet heat olive oil

3. Pour 1/2 of the batter and cook each pancake for 5-10 minutes per side

4. When ready remove from heat and serve

Banana Pancakes

INGREDIENTS

- 2 cup mashed banana
- 2 fresh eggs
- 2 cup milk
- 2 cup whole wheat flour
- 1/2 tsp baking soda
- 1/2 tsp baking powder

DIRECTIONS

1. In a bowl combine all ingredients together and mix well

2. In a skillet heat olive oil

3. Pour 1/2 of the batter and cook each pancake for 5-10 minutes per side

4. When ready remove from heat and serve

Strawberry Muffins

INGREDIENTS

- 1/2 tsp baking soda
- 2 tsp cinnamon
- 2 cup strawberries
- 2 fresh eggs
- 2 tablespoon olive oil
- 2 cup milk
- 2 cups whole wheat flour
- 2 tsp baking soda

DIRECTIONS

1. In a bowl combine all wet ingredients

2. In another bowl combine all dry ingredients

3. Combine wet and dry ingredients together

4. Fold in strawberries and mix well

5. Pour mixture into 25-30 prepared muffin cups, fill 1/2 of the cups

6. Bake for 25-30 minutes at 490 F

Coconut Muffins

INGREDIENTS

- 2 tsp baking soda
- 1/2 tsp baking soda
- 2 tsp cinnamon
- 2 cup coconut flakes
- 2 fresh eggs
- 2 tablespoon olive oil
- 2 cup milk
- 2 cups whole wheat flour

DIRECTIONS

1. In a bowl combine all wet ingredients

2. In another bowl combine all dry ingredients

3. Combine wet and dry ingredients together

4. Pour mixture into 25-30 prepared muffin cups, fill 1/2 of the cups

5. Bake for 25-30 minutes at 490 F

6. When ready remove from the oven and serve

117

Carrot Muffins

INGREDIENTS

- 2 tsp baking soda
- 1/2 tsp baking soda
- 2 cut carrot
- 2 tsp cinnamon
- 2 fresh eggs
- 2 tablespoon olive oil
- 2 cup milk
- 2 cups whole wheat flour

DIRECTIONS

1. In a bowl combine all wet ingredients

2. In another bowl combine all dry ingredients

3. Combine wet and dry ingredients together

4. Pour mixture into 25-30 prepared muffin cups, fill 1/2 of the cups

5. Bake for 25-30 minutes at 490 F

6. When ready remove from the oven and serve

Beans Omelette

INGREDIENTS

- 1/2 cup cheese
- 1/2 tsp basil
- 2 cup beans
- 2 fresh eggs
- 1/2 tsp salt
- 1/2 tsp black pepper
- 2 tablespoon olive oil

DIRECTIONS

121

1. In a bowl combine all ingredients together and mix well

2. In a skillet heat olive oil and pour the fresh egg mixture

3. Cook for 5-10 minutes per side

4. When ready remove omelette from the skillet and serve

Cabbage Omelette

INGREDIENTS

- 1/2 cup cheese
- 1/2 tsp basil
- 2 cup red onion
- 2 cup cabbage
- 2 fresh eggs
- 1/2 tsp salt
- 1/2 tsp black pepper
- 2 tablespoon olive oil

DIRECTIONS

1. In a bowl combine all ingredients together and mix well

2. In a skillet heat olive oil and pour the fresh egg mixture

3. Cook for 5-10 minutes per side

4. When ready remove omelette from the skillet and serve

Mushroom Omelette

INGREDIENTS

- 1/2 cup cheese

- 1/2 tsp basil

- 2 cup mushrooms

- 2 fresh eggs

- 1/2 tsp salt

- 1/2 tsp black pepper

- 2 tablespoon olive oil

DIRECTIONS

125

1. In a bowl combine all ingredients together and mix well

2. In a skillet heat olive oil and pour the fresh egg mixture

3. Cook for 5-10 minutes per side

4. When ready remove omelette from the skillet and serve

Tomato Omelette

INGREDIENTS

- 1/2 cup cheese
- 1/2 tsp basil
- 2 cup tomatoes
- 2 fresh eggs
- 1/2 tsp salt
- 1/2 tsp black pepper
- 2 tablespoon olive oil

DIRECTIONS

1. In a bowl combine all ingredients together and mix well

2. In a skillet heat olive oil and pour the fresh egg mixture

3. Cook for 5-10 minutes per side

4. When ready remove omelette from the skillet and serve

Hazelnut Tart

INGREDIENTS

- 2 tablespoons syrup

- 1/2 lb. dark chocolate

- 2 oz. butter

- pastry sheets

- 4 oz. brown sugar

- 1/2 lb. hazelnuts

- 250 ml double cream

DIRECTIONS

1. Preheat oven to 450 F, unfold pastry sheets and place them on a baking sheet

2. Toss together all ingredients together and mix well

3. Spread mixture in a single layer on the pastry sheets

4. Before baking decorate with your desired fruits

5. Bake at 450 F for 25-30 minutes or until golden brown

6. When ready remove from the oven and serve

Pear Tart

INGREDIENTS

- 1/2 lb. almonds

- pastry sheets

- 2 tablespoons syrup

- 2 lb. pears

- 2 oz. brown sugar

- 1 lb. flaked almonds

- 1/2 lb. porridge oat

131

- 2 oz. flour

DIRECTIONS

1. Preheat oven to 450 F, unfold pastry sheets and place them on a baking sheet

2. Toss together all ingredients together and mix well

3. Spread mixture in a single layer on the pastry sheets

4. Before baking decorate with your desired fruits

5. Bake at 450 F for 25-30 minutes or until golden brown

6. When ready remove from the oven and serve

Cardamom Tart

INGREDIENTS

- 4-6 pears
- 2 tablespoons lemon juice
- pastry sheets
- CARDAMOM FILLING
- 1 lb. butter
- 1 lb. brown sugar
- 1 lb. almonds
- 1/2 lb. flour
- 4 tsp cardamom
- 2 fresh eggs

DIRECTIONS

1. Preheat oven to 450 F, unfold pastry sheets and place them on a baking sheet

2. Toss together all ingredients together and mix well

3. Spread mixture in a single layer on the pastry sheets

4. Before baking decorate with your desired fruits

5. Bake at 450 F for 25-30 minutes or until golden brown

6. When ready remove from the oven and serve

Apple Tart

INGREDIENTS

- 2 lb. apples
- 270 ml double cream
- 2 fresh eggs
- 2 tsp lemon juice
- 4 oz. brown sugar

DIRECTIONS

1. Preheat oven to 450 F, unfold pastry sheets and place them on a baking sheet

2. Toss together all ingredients together and mix well

3. Spread mixture in a single layer on the pastry sheets

4. Before baking decorate with your desired fruits

5. Bake at 450 F for 25-30 minutes or until golden brown

6. When ready remove from the oven and serve

Peach Pecan Pie

INGREDIENTS

- 4 small fresh egg yolks

- 1/2 cup flour

- 2 tsp vanilla extract

- 4-6 cups peaches

- 2 tablespoon preserves

- 2 cup sugar

DIRECTIONS

1. Line a pie plate or pie form with pastry and cover the edges of the plate depending on your preference

2. In a bowl combine all pie ingredients together and mix well

3. Pour the mixture over the pastry

4. Bake at 450 F for 45-50 minutes or until golden brown

5. When ready remove from the oven and let it rest for 30 minutes

Vanilla Cinnamon Cake

Ingredients

- 2 Heaping tsp Cinnamon

- 1 tsp Baking powder

- 2 Tbsp Ground golden flax meal

- 4 Tbsp Oat bran

- 2 tsp Butter buds

- 2 Fresh egg

- 2 Fresh egg white

- 1 tsp Vanilla

- 1/2 tsp Liquid Splenda

- 4 Tbsp Fat free cream cheese

- 2 pk French Vanilla Splenda

Instructions

1. Beat first five ingredients together until cream cheese is thoroughly mixed.
2. ADuken Diet remaining ingredients and mix well. Pour half of the mixture into a Pyrex or microwavable 1 cup container.
3. Put in microwave on high for about 2 minutes or until top springs back.
4. This make 2 cakes the size of a large
5. cupcake. Or you could microwave it all together.

6. The liquid Splenda has zero carbs. You could use Splenda granules no problem; but that may be 4 carbs.
7. I ground the bran just the slightest bit for this.
8. The flax meal gives it nice texture and is all fiber.
9. The butter buds are not essential; you could aDuken Diet extra cinnamon.

Cheesecake

Ingredients

- 2 tbls Oat Bran Splash of skimmed milk
- 2 tbls Quark

- 2 tbls 0% Total greek yoghurt
- Vanilla extract
- Sweetener to taste

Instructions

1. Moisten the oat bran with the milk and press it into
2. the base of a ramekin dish
3. Mix the rest of the ingredients together, sweeten it and pour into the oatbran base
4. Put it in the fridge for 30 minutes

Chicken Kiev

Ingredient

- Chicken breast,

- Extra low fat laughing cow,

- 1 teaspoon dried parsley

- 1 teaspoon garlic granules,

- Salt and pepper,

- 2 egg

- 2 slices DUKEN DIET bread, crumbed,

- Spray light or similar

Instructions

1. Slice into the chicken breast at the thickest point to
2. make a little pocket, mash the laughing cow cheese
3. with the parsley and garlic until well blended, put it into
4. the 'pocket' close it up with 2 wooden cocktail sticks or tie it with string.
5. Beat the egg, then dip the chicken into it, then dip
6. the chicken into the breadcrumbs, pressing them down lightly all over the chicken, lightly spray the baking tray, put the chicken onto the baking tray cocktail stick side
7. up, lightly spray the chicken with frylight , Bake for 4 0-4 6 mins at 200C. Delicious hot or cold

Easy Eggplant Parmesan

Ingredients

• 2 medium eggplant (aubergine) you can peel them but i prefer mine with peel

• cooking spray

• 4 slices DUKEN DIET bread crumbed

• 2 Tbsp grated Parmesan cheese

• 2 teaspoon garlic powder

• 2 teaspoon dried oregano

• 2 teaspoon dried basil

• 2 egg white(s), lightly beaten sauce

• tin of chopped tomatoes

• 1 teaspoon garlic powder

147

- 1 teaspoon dried oregano

- 1 teaspoon dried basil

- 2 tablespoon tomato puree

- Salt and pepper

- herbs of your choice for the sauce , i like italian seasoning in it

- 1 tspoon sweetener (it gives the sauce a more

rounded flavour,)

- 2 diced onion

- 2 very low fat laughing cow (optional)

Instructions

1. Preheat oven to 4 6 0°F. spray a small baking dish with cooking spray; set aside.
2. make up your tomato sauce, put tomatoes , herbs
3. onions into a pan and cook until softened aDuken Diet tomato
4. puree, 1 tsp sweetener and season to taste with salt 4 8

5. and pepper, you will probably only need half the sauce
6. for the dish but it keeps for several days in the fridge.
7. Combine bread crumbs, Parmesan checse and herbs

8. in a medium-size bowl; take a 1 of the mixture out to use as topping slice eggplant into 2 /2-inch-thick slices.

9. put them in a colander and sprinkle with salt, leave for 25 minutes, then rinse and pat dry with kitchen towels, Dip eggplant first into egg whites and then into bread crumb mixture. Bake eggplant on a nonstick baking sheet until lightly browned, about 25 to 26 minutes, flipping once.

10. Place a layer of eggplant on bottom of prepared baking dish, then aDuken Diet 1 of tomato sauce cheese.

11. Repeat until aubergine is all used , top with the last of the bread crumbs, dot with laughing cow cheese, Bake

12. until cheese is melted and sauce is bubbling, about 25

13. minutes more.

Chicken Parmesan

Ingredients

• Tin of chopped tomatoes

• 2 tablespoon tomato puree

• Salt and pepper

• herbs of your choice for the sauce , i like italian seasoning in it

• 1 spoon sweetener (it gives the sauce a more

rounded flavour,)

• 2 diced onion,

• 2 very low fat laughing cow (optional)

• Nonstick cooking spray

- 2 egg white

- 4 slices DUKEN DIET bread crumbed

- 1 tablespoon grated parmesan cheese,

- 1 teaspoon garlic powder

- 1 teaspoon dried oregano

- 1 teaspoon dried basil

Instructions

1.   Preheat your oven to 400° F and lightly coat a baking dish with nonstick cooking spray.
2.   Make up your tomato sauce, put tomatoes , herbs
3.   onions into a pan and cook until softened , aDuken Diet tomato

153

4.   puree, 1 tsp sweetener and season to taste with salt and pepper, you will probably only need half the sauce

5.   for the dish but it keeps for several days in the fridge

6.   lightly beat the egg white . In another bowl, combine

7.   breadcrumbs, parmesan cheese, garlic powder, oregano, and basil.

8.   put aside 1 of the breadcrumb mixture for the

9.   topping. dip the chicken breast in the egg white and then the breadcrumbs mixture until the chicken is

10.   coated on all sides..

11.   Place the chicken breast in a baking dish and bake

12.   for 25 minutes, turn the chicken breast over and lightly

13.   spray the top with nonstick cooking spray.

14.   Bake for another 2 0-25 minutes or until the chicken is lightly browned and not pink in the middle.

15.   top the chicken breast with tomato sauce and the last of the breadcrumb mix dot with laughing cow cheese.

16.   Bake for another five minutes or until the cheese has

17.   melted.

La Soupe Miraculeuse

- 2 green peppers

- 2 bunch celery

- 4 litres water

- 4 low fat beef cubes) far too many. too salty... use

fewer + taste 4 low fat chicken cubes)

- 4 garlic cloves

- 6 large onions

- 2 or 2 tins peeled tomatoes

- 2 large cabbage head

- 6 carrots

Instructions

1. Peel and cut the veggies into equal size pieces. Put them in a soup pot with LOW FAT stock cubes and cover with water. Let them boil for 25 mins, reduce
2. heat and continue cooking until the veggies are tender.

CPSIA information can be obtained
at www.ICGtesting.com
Printed in the USA
LVHW080216240322
714276LV00012B/731

9 781990 207778